What Happens Next?

DEALING WITH LIFE CHANGES

What Happens When I Have a Serious Allergy?

Amy Wallace

PowerKiDS press

Published in 2025 by The Rosen Publishing Group, Inc.
2544 Clinton Street, Buffalo, NY 14224

First Edition

Editor: Theresa Emminizer
Book Design: Leslie Taylor

Photo Credits: Cover all_about_people/Shutterstock.com; p. 5 WBMUL/Shutterstock.com; p. 7 Karen Sarraga/Shutterstock.com; p.9 New Africa/Shutterstock.com; p. 11 Pepermpron/Shutterstock.com; p.13 karen roach/Shutterstock.com; p.15 Pixel-Shot/Shutterstock.com; p. 16 Jarun Ontakrai/Shutterstock.com; p. 17 Alona Siniehina/Shutterstock.com; p. 19 Andrey_Popov/Shutterstock.com; p. 21 MIA Studio/Shuttertstock.com.

Cataloging-in-Publication Data

Names: Wallace, Amy.
Title: What happens when I have a serious allergy? / Amy Wallace
Description: Buffalo, NY : PowerKids Press, 2025. | Series: What happens next? dealing with life changes| Includes glossary and index.
Identifiers: ISBN 9781725327214 (pbk.) | ISBN 9781725327238 (library bound) | ISBN 9781725327245 (ebook)
Subjects: LCSH: Allergy–Juvenile literature. | Food allergy in children–Juvenile literature.
Classification: LCC RC584.W355 2025 | DDC 616.97–dc23

Manufactured in the United States of America

Some of the images in this book illustrate individuals who are models. The depictions do not imply actual situations or events.

CPSIA Compliance Information: Batch #CSPK25. For Further Information contact Rosen Publishing at 1-800-237-9932.

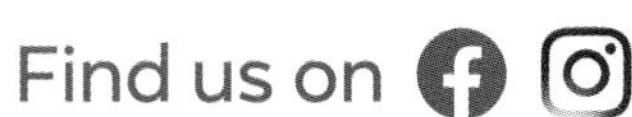

CONTENTS

What Are Allergies?

Allergies are when your body **reacts** badly to certain things around you. These are called allergens. Some people have seasonal allergies. Seasonal allergies might cause you to have itchy eyes or sneeze when certain trees or plants are in bloom. You might have food allergies. Certain foods may cause your skin to itch. You could also have trouble breathing. Or they could make your face, lips, or tongue swell. Or, you might be allergic to other things like dust, pet dander (skin), or bee stings.

Children and adults can have many different types of allergies.

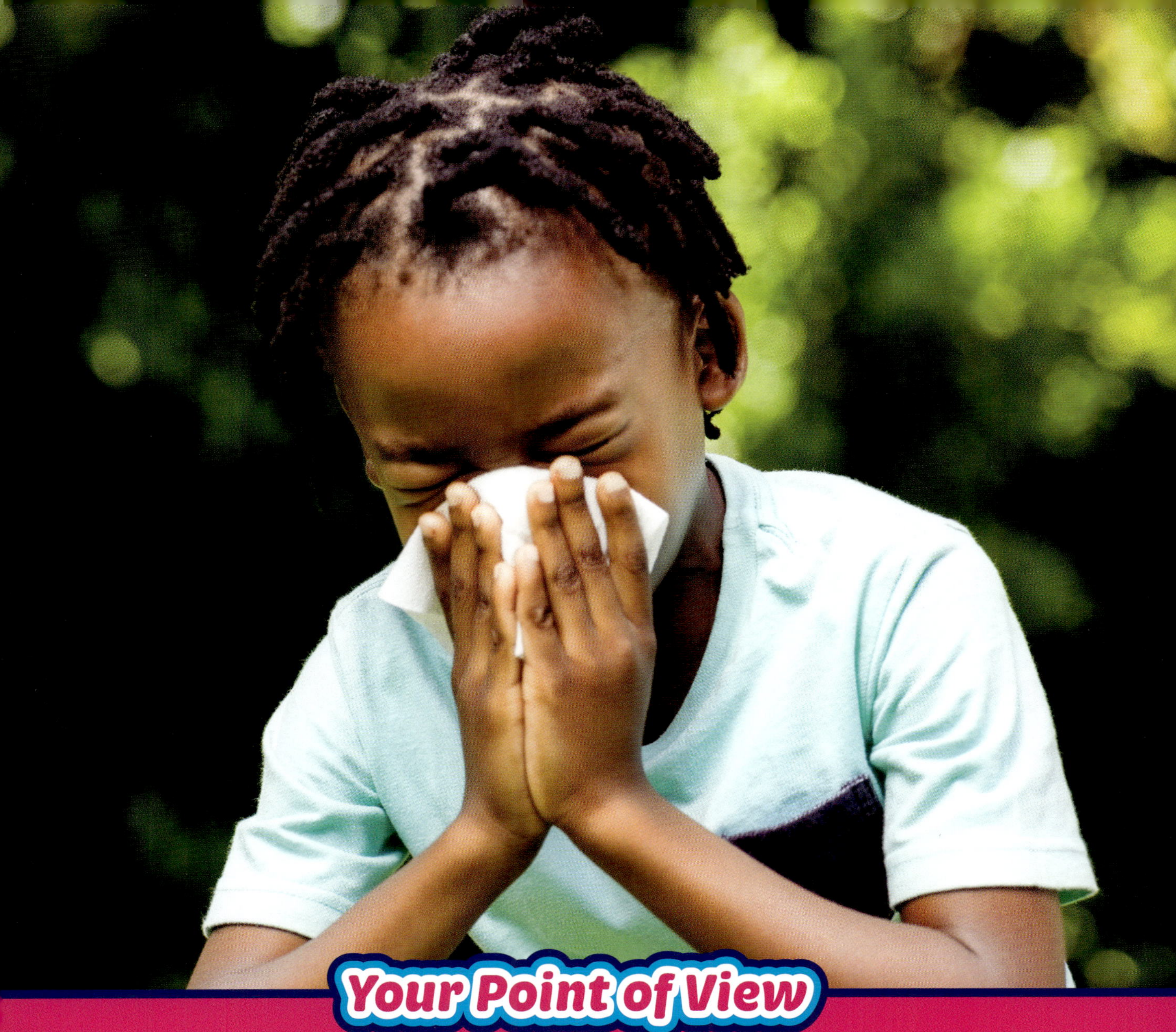

Your Point of View

More than 50 million Americans have different kinds of allergies each year. Allergies are the sixth leading cause of **chronic** illness in the United States.

Food Allergies

You might have a food allergy. Many people are allergic to peanuts, tree nuts, shellfish, dairy, eggs, or fruits. People may be allergic to more than one. These are some of the more common food allergies. However, you can be allergic to any food. There are some people who are allergic to chicken and turkey and others who are allergic to apples. Food allergies occur when your body's immune system sees a certain substance as harmful. It reacts by causing an allergic reaction.

Your Point of View

The immune system is the body system that helps you fight off sickness. The immune system is made up of cells, **tissues**, and **organs** that work together to keep the body safe.

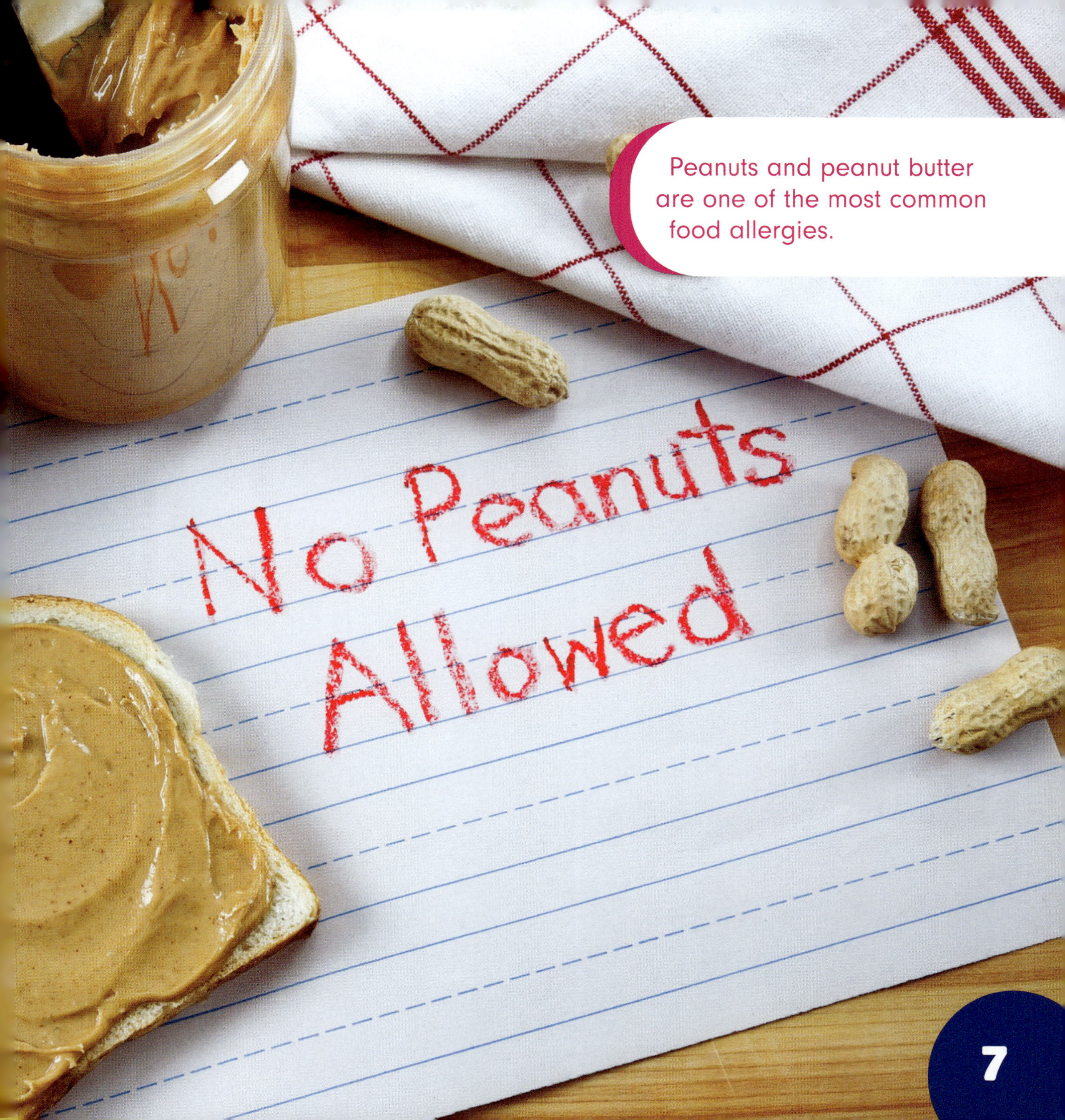

Peanuts and peanut butter are one of the most common food allergies.

Food Intolerance

There's a difference between a food allergy and a food intolerance. An allergic reaction can include getting **hives**, swelling, trouble breathing and throat closing. It's all about the immune system. Food intolerance, however, is when a food causes stomach upset. A food intolerance generally isn't as serious as a food allergy. For example, one kind of food intolerance is lactose intolerance. People who are lactose intolerant often can't have any dairy with the sugar called lactose, or they will end up with an upset stomach.

Do you have a food allergy or a food intolerance? Many people do!

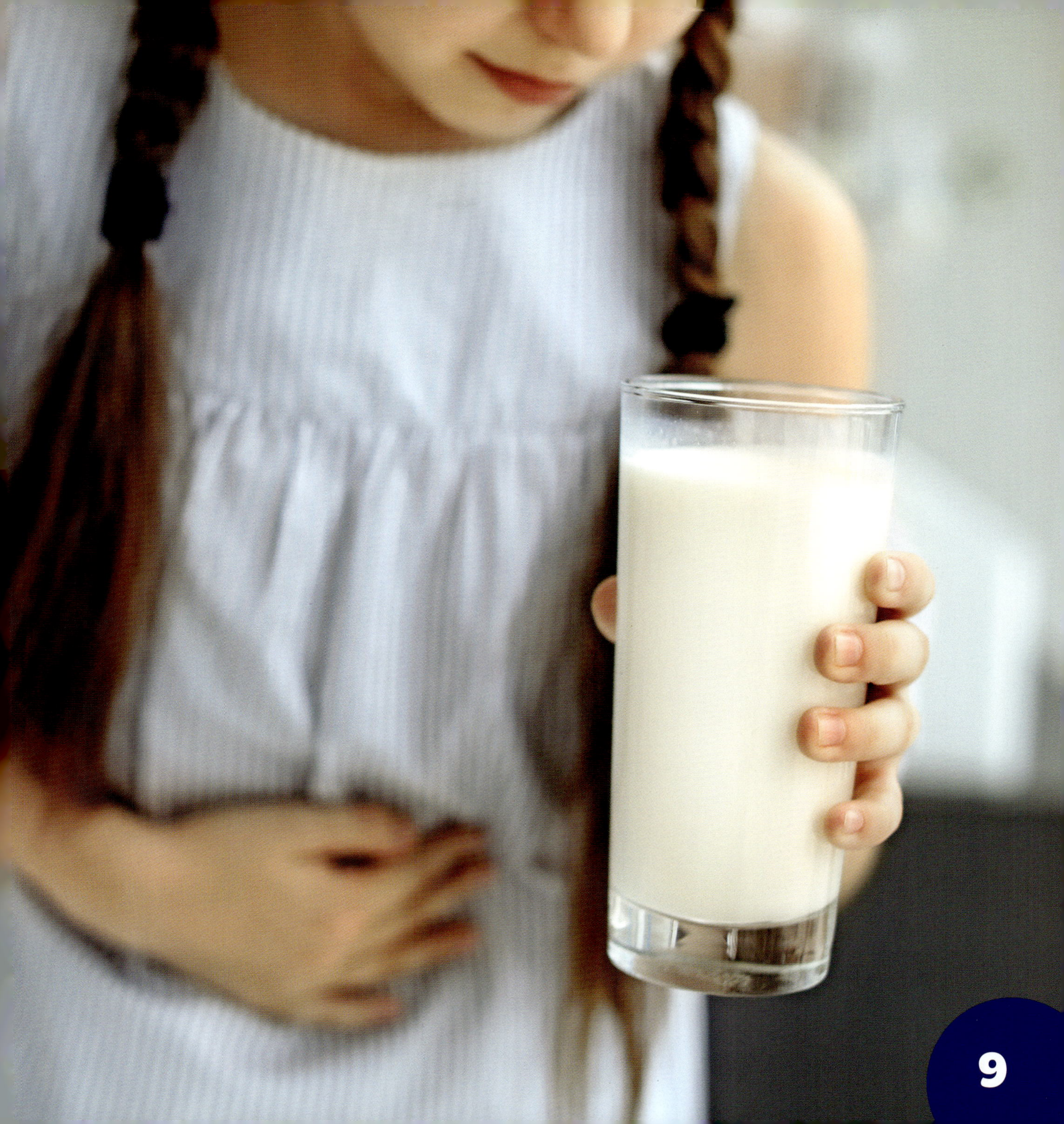

Anaphylaxis

Anaphylaxis is when a person has a severe, or very strong, allergic reaction to a food, insect bite, medicine, or anything else. An anaphylactic reaction is very dangerous. When it happens, the person needs medical treatment right away. Treatment might including a shot of **epinephrine** and a trip to the hospital. If it isn't treated properly, anaphylaxis can be deadly. Anaphylaxis usually involves more than one system of the body at the same time, such as the skin, lungs, or **nervous system**.

Anaphylaxis is a medical emergency, or an event that can be sudden and dangerous and needs fast action. If you think you're having a serious allergic reaction, tell someone quick!

Symptoms of Anaphylaxis

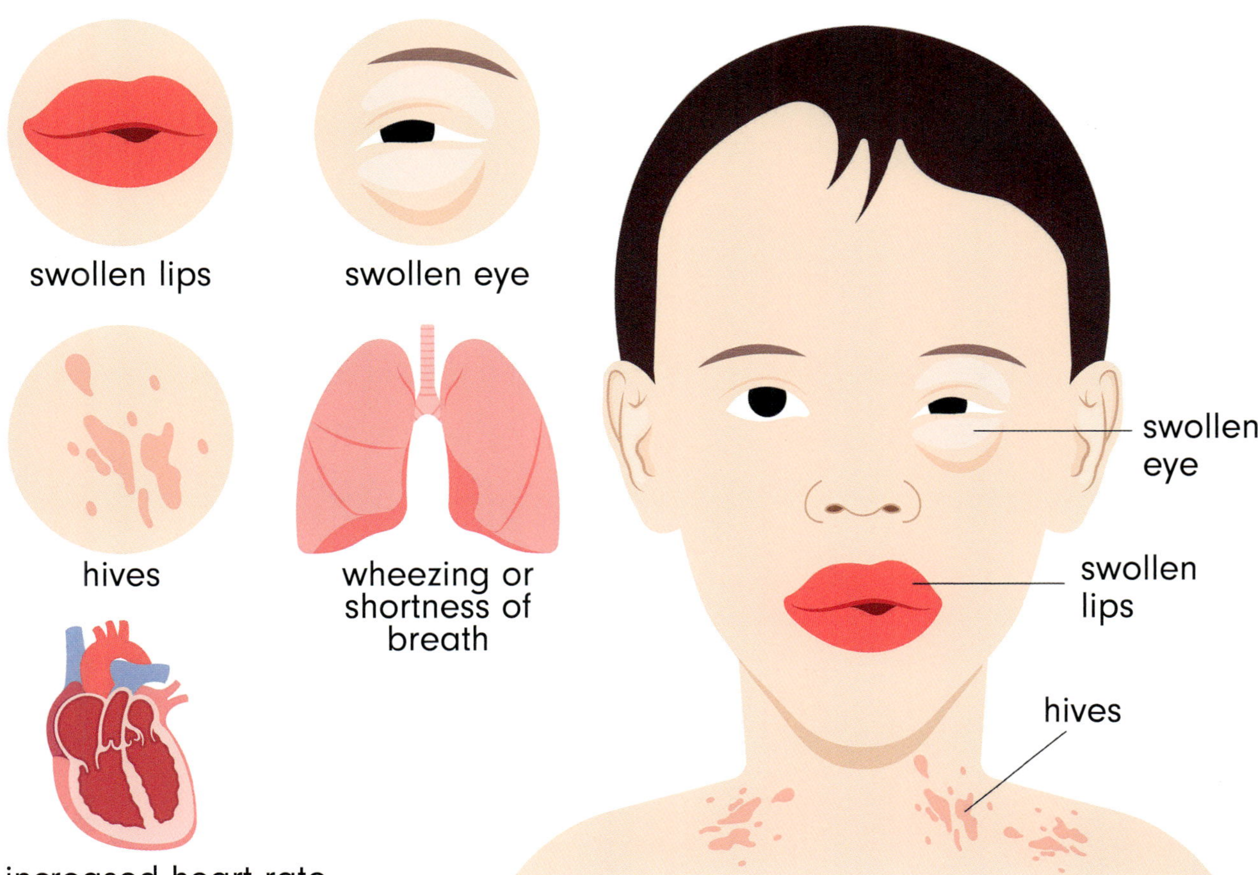

Allergies and School

Going to school when you have serious allergies can be scary. But as allergies have become more common and well known, people in schools have learned to handle them better and keep students safe. Some schools have tables in the cafeteria where only students with food allergies sit. At the allergy tables, certain foods that cause allergic reactions aren't allowed. Teachers may put a sign up on the door of their classroom if a student has an allergy to make sure nobody brings the allergen in.

This classroom has a "Peanut Free Zone" sign on it. Some people have to eat a thing to have an allergic reaction. Some people only have to be around it to have one!

Your Point of View

One in 13 kids has food allergies—that's about two in every U.S. classroom. Everyone can help make sure school is safe for students with food allergies.

Peanut
Free
Zone

What Is an Allergist?

You might not know what's causing your allergic reactions. If that's the case, you'll need to see an allergist! An allergist is a special kind of doctor who **diagnoses** and treats people with allergies. Many people who have allergies also have asthma and eczema. Asthma is a medical condition that causes trouble breathing. Eczema is a skin condition that causes dry skin and itching. If you're diagnosed with an allergy, an allergist will give you medication to treat it.

It's an allergist's job to help you find ways to treat and deal with your allergies!

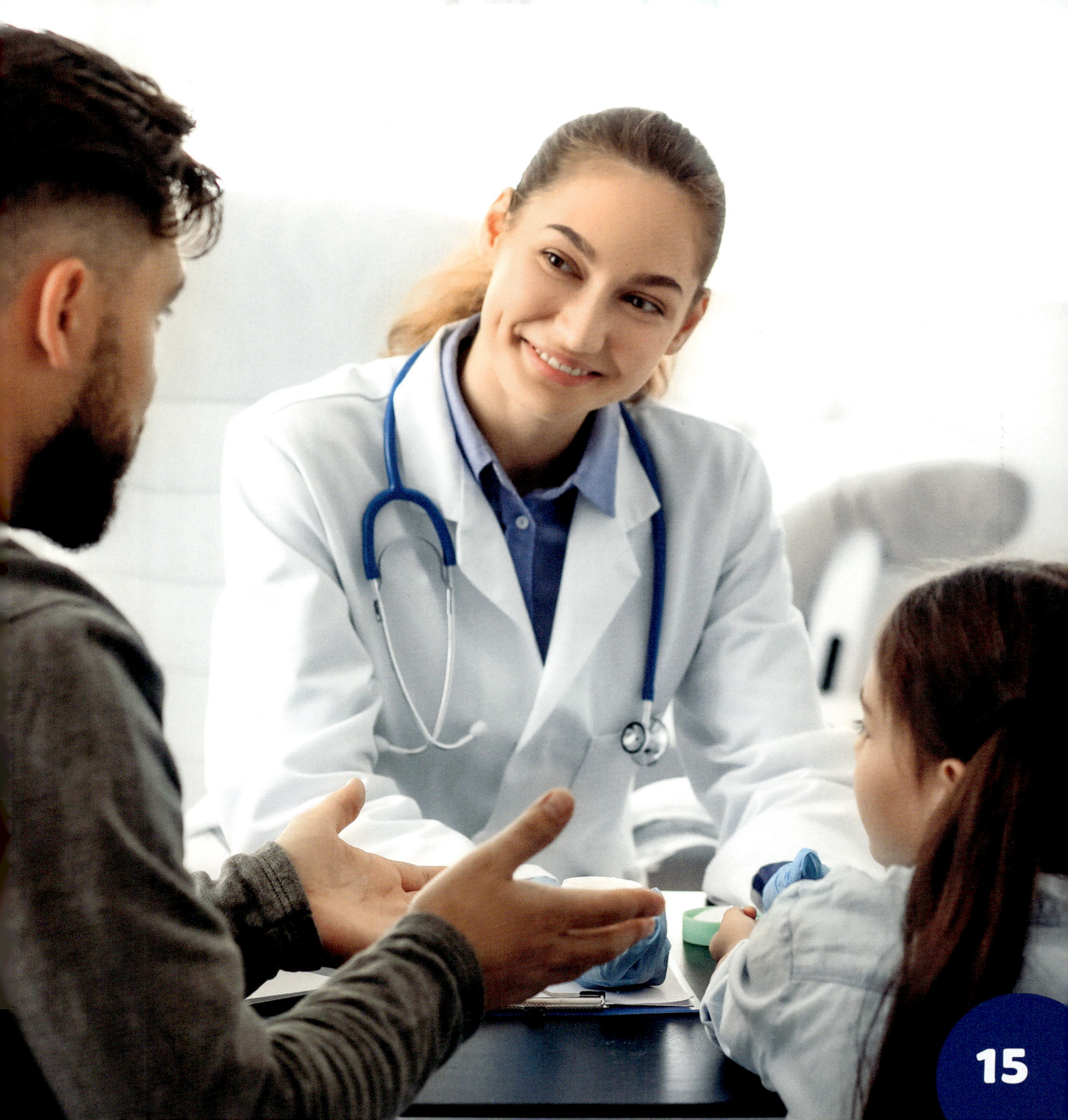

Allergy Testing

There are two main ways to test if a person has an allergy: a skin test and a blood test. During a skin test, a doctor or nurse will prick your skin and add a drop of the suspected, or guessed, allergen to the skin break. The test is usually done on your back or arm. If you are allergic, the skin there will become red and itchy, or you may get hives. Doctors may also test a person's blood to see if they have an allergy.

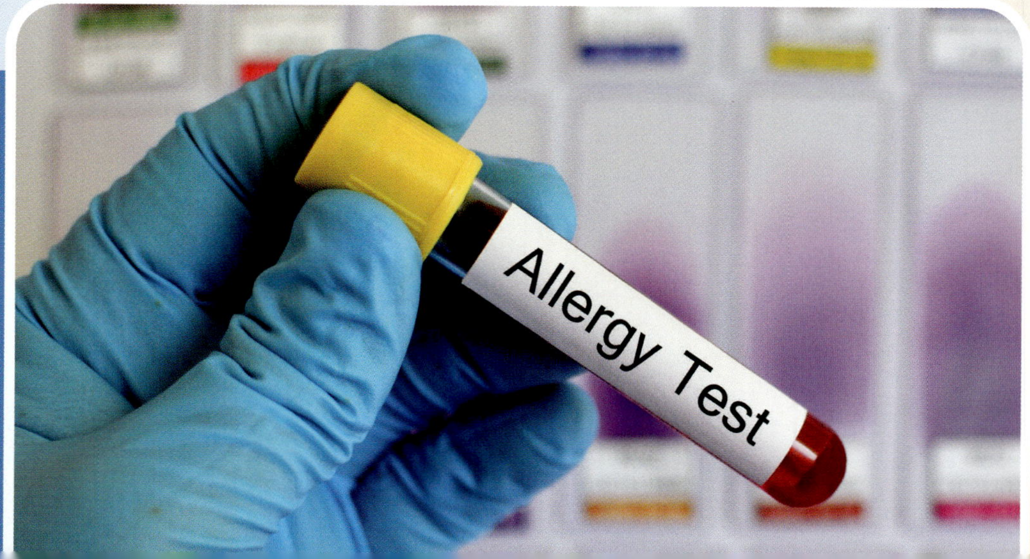

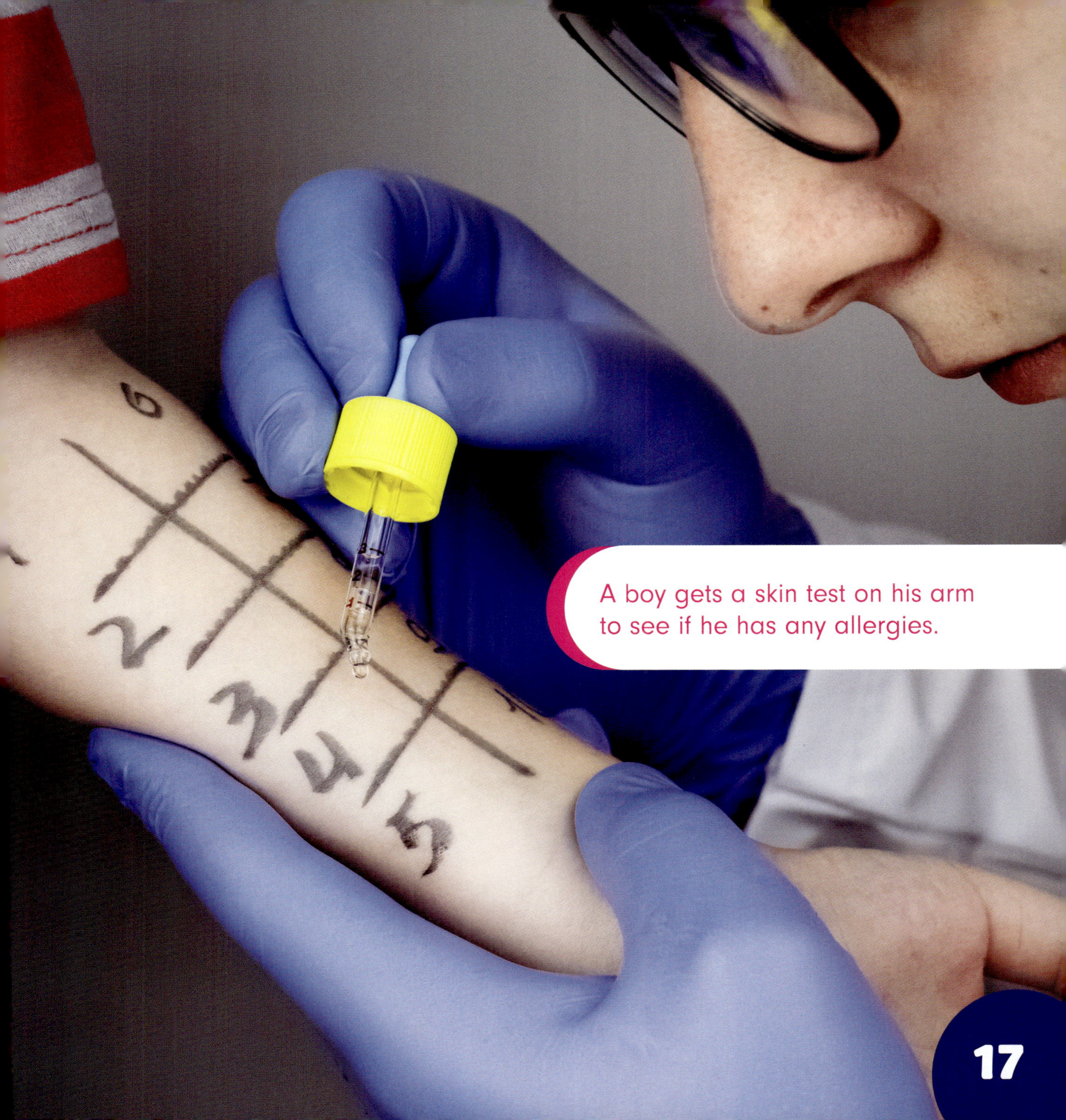

A boy gets a skin test on his arm to see if he has any allergies.

Allergy Treatment

One of the best ways to deal with an allergy is by avoiding, or staying away from, your allergen. If you can't avoid your allergen, though, taking an **antihistamine** like Benadryl can help reverse, or undo, the allergic reaction. If this doesn't work and the symptoms, or signs, are serious, you may have to give yourself a shot with an EpiPen. An EpiPen has a shot of epinephrine that works quickly to reverse the allergic reaction.

An EpiPen should be shot into your outer leg to stop the allergic reaction.

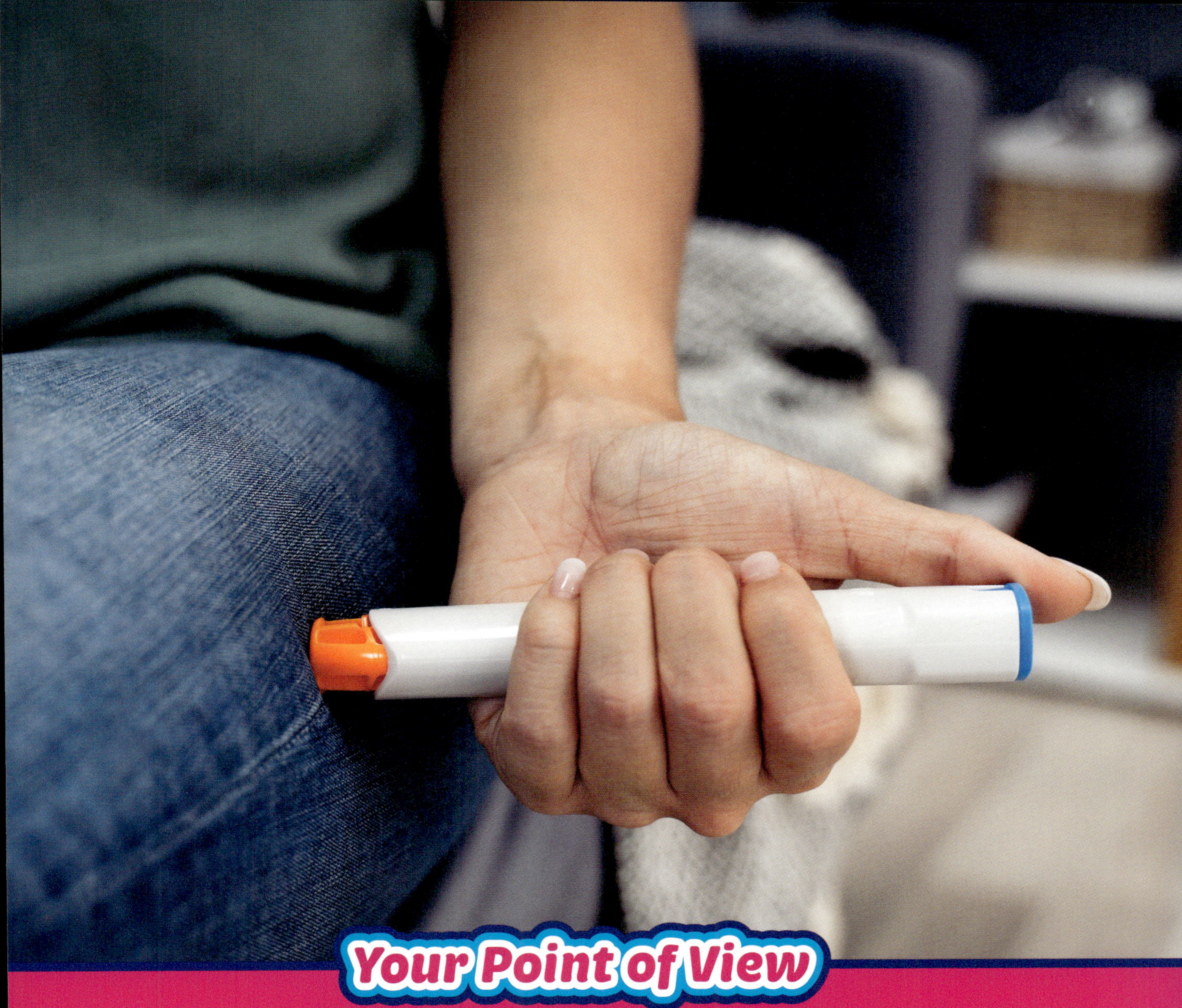

Your Point of View

Epinephrine comes in a premeasured and self-injectable device, or tool. It's the most important medicine to give during a life-threatening, or very dangerous, anaphylaxis attack. People with severe allergies should always have an EpiPen with them.

Taking Control of Your Allergies

If you have an allergy, don't be scared! The first step is to see an allergist and get a diagnosis. They may tell you to avoid your allergen as much as you can and give you medicine. They may help you overcome your allergy through immunotherapy. Immunotherapy involves giving someone bigger and bigger amounts of an allergen to change their immune system's response to it. It can help to carry an antihistamine like Benadryl too. You could also keep an EpiPen with you or at the nurse's office in your school.

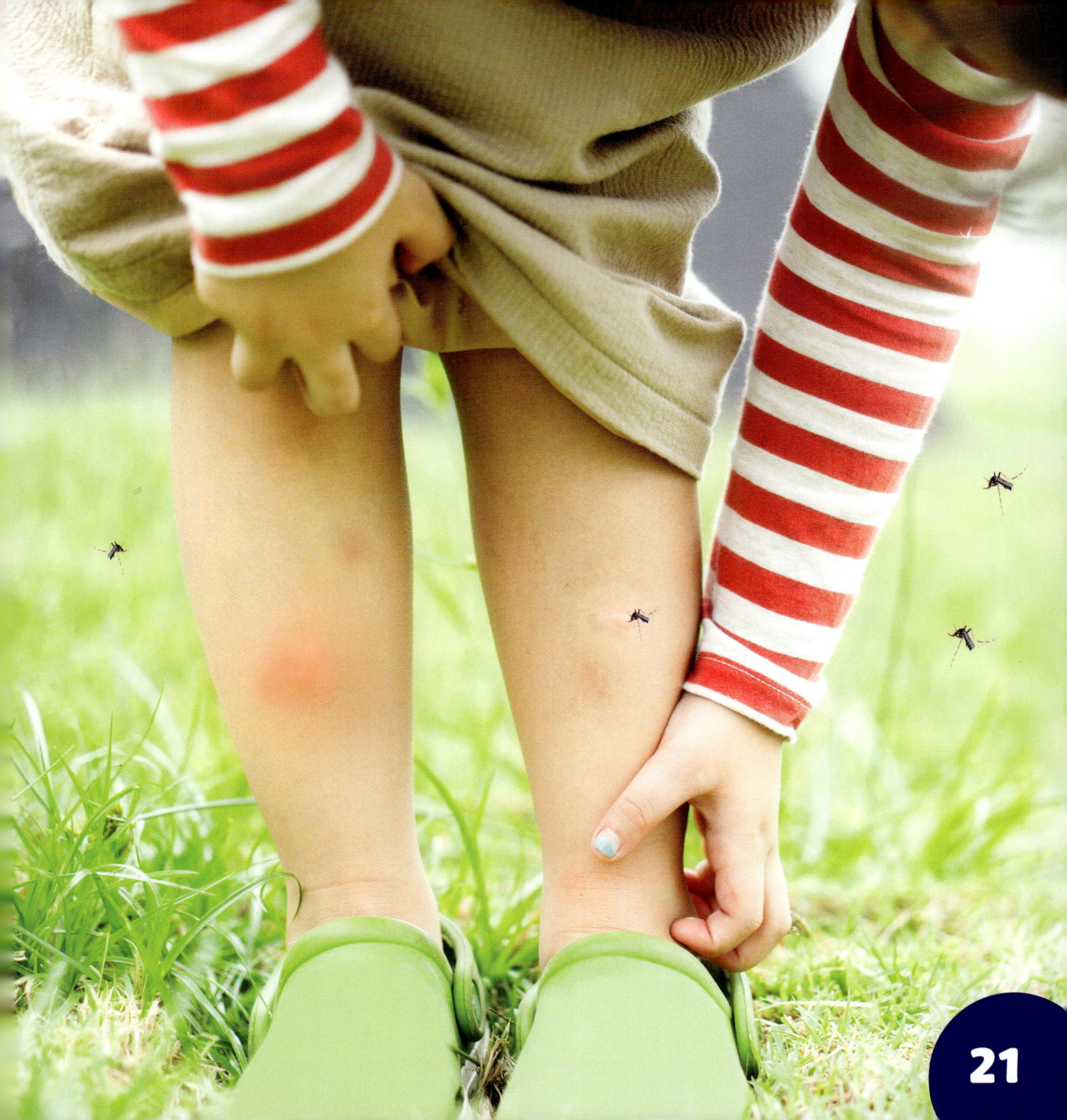

Glossary

antihistamine: A drug used to reverse an allergic reaction.

chronic: Ongoing or happening again and again.

diagnose: To identify or figure out what's making a person sick.

epinephrine: Also known as adrenaline, this is a medicine used to stop anaphylaxis.

hives: An allergic condition in which the skin breaks out in red, itchy patches.

nervous system: The body system that includes the brain, spinal cord, and nerves.

organ: A body part that does a certain task.

react: To respond to something that happens.

tissue: A group of cells of the same kind that come together to form the basic parts that make up a person, plant, or animal.

For More Information

Books

Connors, Kathleen. *I Have a Peanut Allergy*. Buffalo, NY: Enslow Publishing, 2023.

Dickman, Nancy. *Living With Allergies*. Madison, WI: The Creative Company, 2023.

Websites

American Academy of Allergy Asthma and Immunology
www.aaaai.org/conditions-and-treatments/just-for-kids
Play games and read more about life with allergies.

Kids with Food Allergies
www.kidswithfoodallergies.org/
Learn more about living your best life with allergies!

Publisher's note to educators and parents: Our editors have carefully reviewed these websites to ensure that they are suitable for students. Many websites change frequently, however, and we cannot guarantee that a site's future contents will continue to meet our high standards of quality and educational value. Be advised that students should be closely supervised whenever they access the internet.

Index